FIX IT AND FORGET IT

BREAST CANCER

RECIPES

Embracing Healing Through Simplicity, Nourishing Recipes for Strength and Resilience on the Breast Cancer Journey.

MOH LIMS

Copyright © 2023 by Moh Lims

TABLE OF CONTENT

INTRODUCTION

Welcome to a selection of hearty and cozy meals created especially with breast cancer wellness in mind. In order to improve general well-being during the breast cancer journey, eating a healthy, balanced diet is essential.

These "Fix It and Forget It Breast Cancer Recipes" are made to suit the special requirements of those coping with breast cancer by offering not only nourishing and tasty meals, but also dietary guidance.

"Fix It and Forget It" sums up these dishes' main characteristics, which include easiness and simplicity. These recipes are intended to make meal preparation easier for you so that you can concentrate on what really matters—your health and healing—during your treatment and recovery.

This compilation includes a wide range of dishes that highlight foods high in nutrients, such as antioxidants that fight cancer, immune-stimulating substances, and anti-inflammatory qualities.

Every recipe, which ranges from colorful salads to filling main meals and hearty soups and stews, is carefully designed to make mealtime a source of strength and healing.

These dishes are a tribute to the power of food as medicine and the significance of finding joy and sustenance even in trying times, whether you're the one navigating the breast cancer journey or you're supporting a loved one.

Accept the ease of use that comes with Fix It and Forget It, enabling these dishes to serve as a dependable source of care and nourishment while you progress toward wellness. As you set off on your healing road, I'm wishing you courage, solace, and delicious moments.

Sweet and Spicy Roasted Nuts

Ingredients:
- 2 cups mixed nuts (almonds, walnuts, pecans, cashews)
- 2 tablespoons honey
- 1 teaspoon ground cinnamon
- 1/2 teaspoon cayenne pepper
- 1/2 teaspoon sea salt

Instructions:
1. **Preheat the Oven:**
   - Preheat your oven to 350°F (175°C).
2. **Prepare the Nuts:**
   - In a mixing bowl, combine the mixed nuts.
3. **Sweeten with Honey:**
   - Drizzle the honey over the nuts, ensuring they are evenly coated.
4. **Add Spices:**
   - Sprinkle ground cinnamon, cayenne pepper, and sea salt over the nuts. Toss well to coat each nut with the spices.
5. **Spread on a Baking Sheet:**
   - Spread the coated nuts evenly on a parchment-lined baking sheet.
6. **Roast in the Oven:**
   - Roast the nuts in the preheated oven for 12-15 minutes, or until

they become golden brown. Stir the nuts halfway through the baking time for even roasting.

7. **Cooling:**
   - Allow the roasted nuts to cool completely on the baking sheet. They will continue to crisp up as they cool.

8. **Storage:**
   - Once cooled, transfer the sweet and spicy roasted nuts to an airtight container for storage.

Benefits:
1. **Rich in Healthy Fats:**
   - Nuts are a good source of healthy fats, including monounsaturated and polyunsaturated fats, which are beneficial for heart health.

2. **Protein Boost:**
   - Nuts provide a decent amount of protein, making them a satisfying and nutritious snack.

3. **Antioxidant Power:**
   - Honey and nuts contain antioxidants that help combat oxidative stress in the body.

4. **Metabolism Booster:**
   - Cayenne pepper may boost metabolism due to its capsaicin content, potentially aiding in weight management.

5. **Nutrient Variety:**
   - Different nuts bring a variety of nutrients to the mix, including vitamins, minerals, and fiber.

Application:
1. **Snacking:**
   - Enjoy these sweet and spicy roasted nuts as a flavorful and wholesome snack between meals.
2. **Party Appetizer:**
   - Serve these nuts at gatherings or parties as a tasty and health-conscious appetizer.
3. **Salad Topper:**
   - Sprinkle these nuts on top of salads for added crunch and flavor.
4. **Gifts:**
   - Package these roasted nuts in decorative jars or bags for thoughtful and delicious homemade gifts.
5. **Trail Mix:**
   - Combine these nuts with dried fruits and seeds to create a custom trail mix for on-the-go energy.

Berry Chia Pudding

Ingredients:

- 1/2 cup chia seeds
- 2 cups almond milk (or any milk of your choice)
- 1 teaspoon vanilla extract
- 2 tablespoons maple syrup or honey
- 1 cup mixed berries (strawberries, blueberries, raspberries)
- Optional toppings: additional berries, sliced almonds, shredded coconut

Instructions:

1. **Mix Chia Seeds and Liquid:**
   - In a mixing bowl, combine chia seeds, almond milk, vanilla extract, and maple syrup. Stir well to ensure the chia seeds are evenly distributed.

2. **Let it Sit:**
   - Cover the bowl and refrigerate the mixture for at least 4 hours or overnight. The chia seeds will absorb the liquid and create a pudding-like consistency.

3. **Stir Again:**
   - After the initial refrigeration, give the chia pudding a good stir to break up any clumps and promote an even texture.

4. **Add Berries:**
   - Gently fold in the mixed berries, ensuring they are evenly distributed throughout the chia pudding.
5. **Refrigerate Again:**
   - Place the chia pudding back in the refrigerator for at least another hour or until it reaches your desired thickness.
6. **Serve:**
   - Spoon the berry chia pudding into serving bowls or jars.
7. **Top and Enjoy:**
   - Garnish with additional berries, sliced almonds, or shredded coconut. Serve chilled and enjoy!

Benefits:
1. **Omega-3 Fatty Acids:**
   - Chia seeds are rich in omega-3 fatty acids, which are essential for heart health and brain function.
2. **Fiber-Rich:**
   - Chia seeds are an excellent source of fiber, promoting digestive health and helping you feel full for longer.
3. **Antioxidant Boost:**
   - Berries are packed with antioxidants that help combat oxidative stress and inflammation in the body.

4. **Vitamins and Minerals:**
   - Berries contribute essential vitamins and minerals, such as vitamin C and manganese, to support overall health.
5. **Plant-Based Protein:**
   - Chia seeds provide a plant-based source of protein, making this pudding a nutritious and satisfying option.

Application:
1. **Breakfast Option:**
   - Enjoy berry chia pudding as a wholesome and filling breakfast to kickstart your day.
2. **Healthy Dessert:**
   - Serve this pudding as a guilt-free dessert option for those with a sweet tooth.
3. **Snack Time:**
   - Grab a jar of berry chia pudding for a satisfying and nutritious snack during the day.
4. **Post-Workout Fuel:**
   - Replenish your energy and nutrients after a workout with a serving of berry chia pudding.
5. **On-the-Go:**
   - Portion the pudding into small containers for a convenient and portable snack or meal option.

Pomegranate and Walnut Chicken Salad

Ingredients:
- 2 boneless, skinless chicken breasts
- 6 cups mixed salad greens (spinach, arugula, and/or mixed greens)
- 1 cup pomegranate arils (seeds)
- 1/2 cup chopped walnuts, toasted
- 1/2 cup crumbled feta cheese
- 1/4 cup red onion, thinly sliced
- For the dressing:
  - 3 tablespoons extra-virgin olive oil
  - 2 tablespoons balsamic vinegar
  - 1 tablespoon Dijon mustard
  - 1 tablespoon honey
  - Salt and pepper to taste

Instructions:
1. **Cook the Chicken:**
   - Season the chicken breasts with salt and pepper. Grill or pan-cook the chicken until fully cooked, about 6-8 minutes per side. Allow the chicken to rest for a few minutes before slicing it into thin strips.
2. **Prepare the Salad Greens:**
   - In a large salad bowl, combine the mixed greens.
3. **Add Toppings:**
   - Sprinkle pomegranate arils, toasted walnuts, crumbled feta cheese, and

thinly sliced red onion over the salad greens.

4. **Make the Dressing:**
   - In a small bowl, whisk together the olive oil, balsamic vinegar, Dijon mustard, honey, salt, and pepper until well combined.

5. **Assemble the Salad:**
   - Drizzle the dressing over the salad ingredients. Toss gently to coat the greens evenly with the dressing.

6. **Top with Chicken:**
   - Arrange the sliced chicken on top of the salad.

7. **Serve:**
   - Divide the salad among plates and serve immediately.

Benefits:
1. **Lean Protein:**
   - Chicken provides a lean source of protein, essential for muscle maintenance and repair.

2. **Heart-Healthy Fats:**
   - Walnuts contain omega-3 fatty acids, promoting heart health and reducing inflammation.

3. **Antioxidant-Rich:**
   - Pomegranate arils are rich in antioxidants, which help protect cells from damage and support overall health.

4. **Bone Health:**
   - Feta cheese contributes calcium and phosphorus, supporting bone health.
5. **Nutrient Variety:**
   - Mixed greens offer a range of vitamins and minerals, contributing to overall well-being.

Application:
1. **Lunch or Dinner:**
   - Enjoy this chicken salad as a satisfying and nutritious lunch or dinner option.
2. **Entertaining:**
   - Serve this salad at gatherings or dinner parties for a colorful and flavorful dish.
3. **Meal Prep:**
   - Prepare the components ahead of time and assemble the salad just before serving for convenient meal prep.
4. **Holiday Meals:**
   - This festive salad is a great addition to holiday meals, adding a burst of flavor and nutrition to the table.
5. **Picnics or Potlucks:**
   - Pack this salad in a portable container for a refreshing and healthy option at picnics or potlucks.

Eggplant and Tomato Bake

Ingredients:

- 2 large eggplants, sliced into 1/2-inch rounds
- 4 large tomatoes, sliced
- 1 cup shredded mozzarella cheese
- 1/2 cup grated Parmesan cheese
- 2 cloves garlic, minced
- 1/4 cup fresh basil, chopped
- 2 tablespoons olive oil
- Salt and pepper to taste

Instructions:

1. **Preheat the Oven:**
   - Preheat your oven to 375°F (190°C).
2. **Prepare the Eggplant:**
   - Lay out the eggplant slices on a baking sheet. Sprinkle each slice with salt and let them sit for about 15 minutes. This helps draw out excess moisture. After 15 minutes, pat the eggplant slices dry with paper towels.
3. **Assemble the Layers:**
   - In a baking dish, layer the eggplant slices and tomato slices alternately, slightly overlapping.
4. **Make the Cheese Mixture:**

- In a bowl, combine the shredded mozzarella, grated Parmesan, minced garlic, and chopped basil.

5. **Layer the Cheese Mixture:**
   - Sprinkle the cheese mixture evenly over the layered eggplant and tomatoes.

6. **Drizzle with Olive Oil:**
   - Drizzle the olive oil over the top of the cheese layer.

7. **Season:**
   - Season the entire dish with salt and pepper to taste.

8. **Bake:**
   - Bake in the preheated oven for 25-30 minutes or until the cheese is melted and golden brown, and the vegetables are tender.

9. **Serve:**
   - Remove from the oven and let it cool slightly before serving. Garnish with additional fresh basil if desired.

Benefits:

1. **Rich in Antioxidants:**
   - Eggplant and tomatoes are rich in antioxidants, which help protect cells from damage.

2. **Bone Health:**
   - Parmesan cheese contributes calcium and phosphorus, essential for bone health.

3. **Heart-Healthy Fats:**
   - Olive oil provides monounsaturated fats, promoting heart health.
4. **Low in Calories:**
   - This dish is relatively low in calories, making it a healthy option for those watching their calorie intake.

Application:
1. **Side Dish:**
   - Serve the eggplant and tomato bake as a flavorful and nutritious side dish to complement main courses.
2. **Vegetarian Main Course:**
   - This dish can be a satisfying main course for vegetarian meals, offering a hearty and flavorful option.
3. **Potluck or Buffet:**
   - Bring this bake to potlucks or buffets as a colorful and delicious contribution.
4. **Meal Prep:**
   - Prepare this dish ahead of time for meal prep and enjoy it as a quick and convenient meal during the week.
5. **Mediterranean Cuisine:**
   - Incorporate this dish into a Mediterranean-inspired meal by

serving it alongside other dishes like Greek salad and hummus.

Turkey and Vegetable Skillet

Ingredients:

- 1 lb ground turkey
- 2 tablespoons olive oil
- 1 onion, diced
- 2 bell peppers (any color), diced
- 2 zucchini, diced
- 2 cloves garlic, minced
- 1 teaspoon ground cumin
- 1 teaspoon paprika
- 1/2 teaspoon chili powder
- Salt and pepper to taste
- 1 cup cherry tomatoes, halved
- Fresh cilantro or parsley for garnish

Instructions:

1. **Cook the Turkey:**
   - In a large skillet, heat olive oil over medium heat. Add ground turkey and cook until browned, breaking it apart with a spatula as it cooks.

2. **Add Aromatics:**
   - Add diced onion and minced garlic to the skillet. Sauté until the onion is translucent and the garlic is fragrant.

3. **Vegetable Addition:**
   - Add diced bell peppers and zucchini to the skillet. Cook until the vegetables are tender yet still slightly crisp.

4. **Season:**
   - Sprinkle ground cumin, paprika, chili powder, salt, and pepper over the turkey and vegetables. Stir well to evenly coat everything with the spices.
5. **Tomatoes and Finish:**
   - Toss in halved cherry tomatoes and cook for an additional 2-3 minutes, just until the tomatoes are slightly softened.
6. **Garnish and Serve:**
   - Remove the skillet from heat. Garnish with fresh cilantro or parsley. Serve the turkey and vegetable skillet over rice, quinoa, or your favorite grain.

Benefits:
1. **Lean Protein:**
   - Turkey is a lean source of protein, supporting muscle health and providing essential amino acids.
2. **Vegetable Nutrients:**
   - Bell peppers, zucchini, and tomatoes are rich in vitamins, minerals, and antioxidants, promoting overall health.
3. **Heart-Healthy Fats:**
   - Olive oil contributes monounsaturated fats, which are beneficial for heart health.

4. **Low Carb Option:**
   - This recipe is relatively low in carbohydrates, making it suitable for low-carb or keto diets.

Application:

1. **Quick Weeknight Dinner:**
   - The turkey and vegetable skillet is a quick and easy recipe, perfect for busy weeknight dinners.
2. **Meal Prep:**
   - Prepare a batch and divide it into containers for a convenient and healthy meal prep option for the week.
3. **Taco Filling:**
   - Use the seasoned turkey and vegetable mixture as a flavorful filling for tacos or burritos.
4. **Wrap or Burrito Bowl:**
   - Create wraps or burrito bowls by serving the turkey and vegetables with tortillas or over a bed of rice or quinoa.
5. **Versatile Base:**
   - Customize the recipe by adding your favorite vegetables or adjusting the spices to suit your taste preferences.

Broccoli and Almond Soup

Ingredients:

- 1 lb broccoli florets
- 1 cup almonds, blanched and slivered
- 1 onion, diced
- 2 cloves garlic, minced
- 4 cups vegetable broth
- 1 cup unsweetened almond milk
- 2 tablespoons olive oil
- Salt and pepper to taste
- Lemon wedges for serving (optional)

Instructions:

1. **Blanch Almonds:**
   - In a pot of boiling water, blanch the almonds for 1-2 minutes, then drain and rinse with cold water. Peel the almonds and sliver them.

2. **Sauté Aromatics:**
   - In a large soup pot, heat olive oil over medium heat. Add diced onion and minced garlic. Sauté until the onion is translucent and the garlic is fragrant.

3. **Add Broccoli and Almonds:**
   - Add broccoli florets and slivered almonds to the pot. Cook for 2-3 minutes, stirring occasionally.

4. **Vegetable Broth:**
   - Pour in the vegetable broth, bringing the mixture to a boil.

Reduce the heat to low, cover, and simmer for about 15-20 minutes or until the broccoli is tender.

5. **Blend the Soup:**
   - Use an immersion blender or transfer the soup to a blender (in batches) to puree until smooth. Be cautious when blending hot liquids.

6. **Add Almond Milk:**
   - Return the soup to the pot and stir in the unsweetened almond milk. Simmer for an additional 5 minutes.

7. **Season:**
   - Season the soup with salt and pepper to taste. Adjust the consistency by adding more almond milk or vegetable broth if desired.

8. **Serve:**
   - Ladle the soup into bowls. Squeeze a bit of lemon juice over each serving for added freshness (optional).

Benefits:
1. **Nutrient-Rich:**
   - Broccoli is a good source of vitamins C and K, fiber, and antioxidants.

2. **Heart-Healthy Fats:**
   - Almonds provide monounsaturated fats, which are beneficial for heart health.

3. **Dairy-Free and Vegan:**
   - This soup is dairy-free and vegan, making it suitable for those with dietary restrictions.
4. **Bone Health:**
   - Broccoli and almonds contribute to bone health by providing calcium and vitamin K.

Application:
1. **Light Lunch or Dinner:**
   - Enjoy this soup as a light and nutritious lunch or dinner option.
2. **Appetizer:**
   - Serve smaller portions as an appetizer before a main course.
3. **Meal Prep:**
   - Make a large batch and store it in individual portions for convenient meal prep throughout the week.
4. **Cold Weather Comfort:**
   - Warm up on chilly days with a comforting bowl of broccoli and almond soup.
5. **Garnish and Customize:**
   - Garnish with additional slivered almonds or fresh herbs for added texture and flavor. Customize the soup by adding spices like cumin or coriander according to your taste preferences.

Quinoa and Black Bean Bowl

Ingredients:

- 1 cup quinoa, rinsed
- 2 cups water or vegetable broth
- 1 can (15 oz) black beans, drained and rinsed
- 1 cup corn kernels (fresh, frozen, or canned)
- 1 red bell pepper, diced
- 1 avocado, sliced
- 1 lime, juiced
- 1/4 cup fresh cilantro, chopped
- 1 teaspoon ground cumin
- 1 teaspoon chili powder
- Salt and pepper to taste
- Optional toppings: salsa, Greek yogurt, shredded cheese

Instructions:

1. **Cook Quinoa:**
   - In a medium saucepan, combine quinoa and water or vegetable broth. Bring to a boil, then reduce heat to low, cover, and simmer for 15-20 minutes or until quinoa is cooked and water is absorbed.

2. **Prepare Black Beans:**
   - While quinoa is cooking, heat black beans in a small saucepan over medium heat. Stir in ground cumin,

chili powder, salt, and pepper. Cook until heated through.

3. **Cook Corn and Bell Pepper:**
   - In a separate pan, sauté corn kernels and diced red bell pepper until they are tender-crisp, about 5 minutes.

4. **Assemble the Bowl:**
   - In serving bowls, layer cooked quinoa, seasoned black beans, sautéed corn and bell pepper, sliced avocado, and chopped cilantro.

5. **Squeeze Lime:**
   - Drizzle lime juice over the bowl for a burst of freshness.

6. **Add Toppings:**
   - Optional: Top the bowl with salsa, a dollop of Greek yogurt, or shredded cheese.

7. **Mix and Serve:**
   - Gently toss the ingredients together in the bowl. Serve immediately.

Benefits:

1. **Complete Protein:**
   - Quinoa and black beans together form a complete protein, providing all nine essential amino acids.

2. **Rich in Fiber:**
   - Black beans and quinoa are both excellent sources of fiber, promoting digestive health.

3. **Vitamins and Antioxidants:**
   - Red bell pepper and avocado contribute vitamins A and C, along with antioxidants.
4. **Heart-Healthy Fats:**
   - Avocado provides monounsaturated fats, supporting heart health.

Application:

1. **Quick and Healthy Dinner:**
   - Enjoy this quinoa and black bean bowl as a quick, healthy, and satisfying dinner option.
2. **Lunchbox Meal:**
   - Pack this bowl for a nutritious and filling lunch. Keep ingredients separate and assemble before eating for freshness.
3. **Meatless Monday Option:**
   - This plant-based bowl is an excellent choice for Meatless Monday or as part of a vegetarian/vegan meal plan.
4. **Customizable:**
   - Customize the bowl with your favorite toppings, such as salsa, Greek yogurt, or cheese.
5. **Meal Prep:**
   - Make a big batch of quinoa, black beans, and sautéed veggies at the beginning of the week for easy assembly on busy days.

Mango and Avocado Salad

Ingredients:

- 2 ripe mangoes, peeled and diced
- 2 ripe avocados, peeled, pitted, and diced
- 1/2 red onion, finely sliced
- 1 cup cherry tomatoes, halved
- 1/4 cup fresh cilantro, chopped
- Juice of 2 limes
- 2 tablespoons extra-virgin olive oil
- Salt and pepper to taste
- Optional: 1 jalapeño, finely diced (for a spicy kick)

Instructions:

1. **Prepare the Ingredients:**
   - Dice the mangoes and avocados into bite-sized pieces. Finely slice the red onion, halve the cherry tomatoes, and chop the cilantro.

2. **Combine Ingredients:**
   - In a large mixing bowl, combine the diced mangoes, avocados, sliced red onion, cherry tomatoes, and chopped cilantro.

3. **Make the Dressing:**
   - In a small bowl, whisk together the lime juice, extra-virgin olive oil, salt, and pepper. Optional: Add diced jalapeño for a spicy kick.

4. **Dress the Salad:**
   - Pour the dressing over the salad ingredients and gently toss to coat evenly.
5. **Chill (Optional):**
   - Allow the salad to chill in the refrigerator for 15-30 minutes to enhance the flavors.
6. **Serve:**
   - Serve the mango and avocado salad in a large bowl or divide it into individual servings.

Benefits:
1. **Vitamins and Antioxidants:**
   - Mangoes are rich in vitamins A and C, while avocados contribute vitamin K, E, and various antioxidants.
2. **Heart-Healthy Fats:**
   - Avocados provide monounsaturated fats, which are beneficial for heart health.
3. **Hydration:**
   - Mangoes have high water content, contributing to hydration.
4. **Digestive Health:**
   - The fiber in mangoes and avocados supports healthy digestion.

Application:
1. **Refreshing Side Dish:**
   - Serve the mango and avocado salad as a refreshing side dish alongside grilled chicken, fish, or your favorite protein.
2. **Summer Picnic or BBQ:**
   - This vibrant salad is perfect for summer picnics, barbecues, or outdoor gatherings.
3. **Taco or Burrito Filling:**
   - Use the salad as a filling for tacos or burritos to add a burst of freshness and flavor.
4. **Lunchbox Salad:**
   - Pack this salad in a lunchbox for a nutritious and energizing meal.
5. **Cinco de Mayo Celebration:**
   - Include this salad in your Cinco de Mayo celebration for a tropical and festive touch.

Cauliflower Rice Stir-Fry

Ingredients:

- 1 medium-sized cauliflower, grated or processed into rice-sized pieces
- 2 tablespoons sesame oil or olive oil
- 1 cup mixed vegetables (carrots, bell peppers, peas, broccoli, etc.), chopped
- 2 cloves garlic, minced
- 1-inch piece of ginger, grated
- 1 cup cooked protein (tofu, chicken, shrimp, or your choice)
- 3 tablespoons soy sauce or tamari (for a gluten-free option)
- 1 tablespoon oyster sauce (optional)
- 2 green onions, chopped
- Sesame seeds for garnish
- Salt and pepper to taste

Instructions:

1. **Prepare Cauliflower Rice:**
   - Grate the cauliflower or process it in a food processor until it resembles rice-sized grains.

2. **Stir-Fry Vegetables:**
   - Heat oil in a large wok or skillet over medium-high heat. Add minced garlic and grated ginger, stirring for about 30 seconds until fragrant.

3. **Add Vegetables:**
   - Add the mixed vegetables to the wok. Stir-fry for 3-5 minutes until

they are slightly tender but still crisp.

4. **Cook Cauliflower Rice:**
   - Push the vegetables to one side of the wok and add the grated cauliflower. Stir-fry for an additional 3-5 minutes until the cauliflower is tender but not mushy.

5. **Protein Addition:**
   - Push the cauliflower rice to the side and add the cooked protein (tofu, chicken, shrimp, etc.) to the empty space. Stir until the protein is heated through.

6. **Combine and Season:**
   - Mix everything together in the wok. Pour soy sauce (or tamari) and oyster sauce (if using) over the stir-fry. Toss well to coat all ingredients evenly.

7. **Adjust Seasoning:**
   - Taste the stir-fry and adjust the seasoning with salt and pepper as needed.

8. **Finish and Garnish:**
   - Remove the wok from heat. Stir in chopped green onions. Garnish with sesame seeds.

9. **Serve:**
   - Serve the cauliflower rice stir-fry hot, either on its own or as a side dish.

Benefits:
1. **Low-Carb Alternative:**
   - Cauliflower rice is a low-carb alternative to traditional rice, making this stir-fry suitable for low-carb or keto diets.
2. **Rich in Vegetables:**
   - The stir-fry is packed with a variety of colorful vegetables, providing essential vitamins, minerals, and antioxidants.
3. **Versatile Protein Options:**
   - This recipe accommodates various protein choices, allowing flexibility for different dietary preferences.
4. **Fiber Content:**
   - Cauliflower and vegetables contribute dietary fiber, supporting digestive health.

Application:
1. **Quick Weeknight Dinner:**
   - This cauliflower rice stir-fry is a quick and healthy option for a satisfying weeknight dinner.

2. **Meal Prep:**
   - Prepare a large batch and portion it into containers for easy meal prep throughout the week.
3. **Vegetarian or Vegan Meal:**
   - Skip the animal protein or use plant-based alternatives to make this stir-fry a vegetarian or vegan-friendly dish.
4. **Customizable:**
   - Customize the stir-fry by adding your favorite vegetables, adjusting the level of spiciness, or experimenting with different sauces.
5. **Asian-Inspired Menu:**
   - Include this dish as part of an Asian-inspired menu, serving it alongside other favorites like spring rolls or dumplings.

Grilled Vegetable Skewers

Ingredients:

- 1 zucchini, sliced into rounds
- 1 yellow bell pepper, cut into chunks
- 1 red onion, cut into wedges
- 1 pint cherry tomatoes
- 8-10 button mushrooms, cleaned
- 2 tablespoons olive oil
- 2 cloves garlic, minced
- 1 teaspoon dried oregano
- 1 teaspoon dried thyme
- Salt and pepper to taste
- Wooden or metal skewers

Instructions:

1. **Prep the Vegetables:**
   - Clean and cut the vegetables into bite-sized pieces.
2. **Marinate Vegetables:**
   - In a bowl, combine olive oil, minced garlic, dried oregano, dried thyme, salt, and pepper. Toss the vegetables in the marinade, ensuring they are well-coated. Let them marinate for at least 15-30 minutes.
3. **Skewer the Vegetables:**
   - Thread the marinated vegetables onto skewers, alternating the different types to create colorful and varied skewers.

4. **Preheat the Grill:**
   - Preheat your grill to medium-high heat.
5. **Grill the Skewers:**
   - Place the vegetable skewers on the preheated grill. Grill for about 10-15 minutes, turning occasionally, until the vegetables are tender and have a nice char.
6. **Baste with Marinade:**
   - Occasionally baste the skewers with the remaining marinade to add flavor and prevent them from drying out.
7. **Check for Doneness:**
   - Test for doneness by inserting a fork into the vegetables. They should be tender but not mushy.
8. **Serve:**
   - Remove the skewers from the grill and serve immediately.

Benefits:
1. **Rich in Nutrients:**
   - The variety of vegetables provides a range of essential vitamins, minerals, and antioxidants.
2. **Low in Calories:**
   - Grilled vegetable skewers are a low-calorie and nutritious option, suitable for those watching their calorie intake.

3. **Fiber-Rich:**
   - Vegetables are high in dietary fiber, promoting digestive health and providing a feeling of fullness.
4. **Heart-Healthy:**
   - Olive oil used in the marinade contains monounsaturated fats, which are beneficial for heart health.

Application:
1. **Summer BBQ:**
   - Grilled vegetable skewers are a perfect addition to summer barbecues, offering a healthy and colorful alternative to traditional BBQ fare.
2. **Side Dish:**
   - Serve the skewers as a flavorful and nutritious side dish alongside grilled meats or fish.
3. **Vegetarian Main Course:**
   - These skewers can be a delicious vegetarian main course. Serve them over quinoa, couscous, or a bed of greens for a complete meal.
4. **Party Appetizer:**
   - Make mini skewers for a party or gathering as a delightful and visually appealing appetizer.

5. **Meal Prep:**
   - Prepare a batch of grilled vegetable skewers and store them in the refrigerator for quick and convenient meal prep during the week.

Greek Yogurt Parfait

Ingredients:
- 1 cup Greek yogurt (plain or flavored)
- 1 cup mixed berries (strawberries, blueberries, raspberries)
- 1/2 cup granola
- 1 tablespoon honey or maple syrup
- 1/4 cup nuts (almonds, walnuts, or your choice), chopped
- Optional: 1 teaspoon chia seeds or flaxseeds

Instructions:
1. **Layer the Greek Yogurt:**
   - Start by spooning a layer of Greek yogurt into the bottom of a glass or a bowl.
2. **Add Berries:**
   - Layer a portion of mixed berries on top of the Greek yogurt.
3. **Sprinkle Granola:**
   - Sprinkle a layer of granola over the berries. This adds crunch and additional fiber.
4. **Drizzle with Honey:**
   - Drizzle honey or maple syrup over the granola layer for sweetness.
5. **Repeat Layers:**
   - Repeat the layers until you fill the glass or bowl, finishing with a final drizzle of honey on top.

6. **Top with Nuts and Seeds:**
   - Sprinkle chopped nuts over the parfait. Optionally, add chia seeds or flaxseeds for added nutritional benefits.
7. **Serve:**
   - Serve the Greek Yogurt Parfait immediately and enjoy!

Benefits:
1. **Protein-Rich:**
   - Greek yogurt is an excellent source of protein, which helps keep you full and supports muscle health.
2. **Antioxidants:**
   - Berries are rich in antioxidants, which help protect cells from damage caused by free radicals.
3. **Fiber-Packed:**
   - Granola and berries contribute dietary fiber, promoting digestive health.
4. **Healthy Fats:**
   - Nuts provide healthy fats, contributing to heart health and satiety.
5. **Vitamins and Minerals:**
   - Berries and nuts offer a variety of essential vitamins and minerals.

Application:

1. **Breakfast Option:**
   - Greek Yogurt Parfait makes for a delicious and nutritious breakfast option, providing a good balance of protein, fiber, and vitamins.
2. **Snack Time:**
   - Enjoy it as a satisfying and healthy snack between meals.
3. **Dessert Alternative:**
   - Serve Greek Yogurt Parfait as a lighter and healthier dessert alternative.
4. **Post-Workout Refuel:**
   - The combination of protein and carbohydrates makes it a suitable option for post-workout recovery.
5. **Customizable:**
   - Customize the parfait by adding your favorite fruits, switching up the yogurt flavor, or incorporating different types of nuts and seeds.

Turmeric-Ginger Carrot Soup

Ingredients:

- 1 lb carrots, peeled and chopped
- 1 onion, diced
- 3 cloves garlic, minced
- 1-inch piece of ginger, grated
- 1 teaspoon ground turmeric
- 1/2 teaspoon ground cumin
- 1/2 teaspoon ground coriander
- 4 cups vegetable broth
- 1 can (13.5 oz) coconut milk
- 2 tablespoons olive oil
- Salt and pepper to taste
- Fresh cilantro or parsley for garnish (optional)

Instructions:

1. **Sauté Aromatics:**
   - In a large pot, heat olive oil over medium heat. Add diced onion, minced garlic, and grated ginger. Sauté until the onion is translucent and the aromatics are fragrant.
2. **Add Carrots and Spices:**
   - Add the chopped carrots to the pot. Stir in ground turmeric, ground cumin, and ground coriander. Cook for 5 minutes, allowing the spices to coat the carrots.

3. **Pour in Broth:**
   - Pour in the vegetable broth, ensuring that the carrots are fully submerged. Bring the mixture to a boil.

4. **Simmer and Cook:**
   - Reduce the heat to low, cover the pot, and simmer for about 20-25 minutes or until the carrots are tender.

5. **Blend the Soup:**
   - Use an immersion blender to blend the soup until smooth. Alternatively, transfer the soup to a blender in batches, blending until smooth. Be cautious when blending hot liquids.

6. **Add Coconut Milk:**
   - Pour in the coconut milk and stir well. Simmer for an additional 5-7 minutes to allow the flavors to meld.

7. **Season:**
   - Season the soup with salt and pepper to taste. Adjust the seasoning as needed.

8. **Serve:**
   - Ladle the Turmeric-Ginger Carrot Soup into bowls. Garnish with fresh cilantro or parsley if desired.

Benefits:
1. **Anti-Inflammatory Properties:**
   - Turmeric and ginger have anti-inflammatory properties, which may help reduce inflammation in the body.
2. **Rich in Antioxidants:**
   - Carrots are rich in antioxidants, contributing to overall health and well-being.
3. **Immune System Support:**
   - Garlic and ginger are known for their immune-boosting properties.
4. **Heart-Healthy:**
   - Coconut milk provides healthy fats that may support heart health.

Application:
1. **Comforting Meal:**
   - Enjoy Turmeric-Ginger Carrot Soup as a comforting and nutritious meal, especially during colder months.
2. **Lunch or Dinner Option:**
   - Serve the soup as a light lunch or dinner option alongside a salad or crusty bread.
3. **Meal Prep:**
   - Make a large batch and store it in individual portions for convenient meal prep throughout the week.

4. **Anti-Inflammatory Diet:**
   - Incorporate this soup into an anti-inflammatory diet to harness the potential benefits of turmeric and ginger.
5. **Soup Bar:**
   - Feature this vibrant soup at a soup bar or buffet during gatherings or events.

Chickpea and Tomato Salad

Ingredients:
- 2 cans (15 oz each) chickpeas, drained and rinsed
- 1 pint cherry tomatoes, halved
- 1 cucumber, diced
- 1/2 red onion, finely chopped
- 1/4 cup fresh parsley, chopped
- 1/4 cup feta cheese, crumbled (optional)
- 3 tablespoons extra-virgin olive oil
- 2 tablespoons red wine vinegar
- 1 teaspoon dried oregano
- Salt and pepper to taste
- Optional: Kalamata olives for garnish

Instructions:
1. **Prepare Chickpeas:**
   - Drain and rinse the canned chickpeas under cold water.
2. **Combine Ingredients:**
   - In a large bowl, combine the chickpeas, cherry tomatoes, cucumber, red onion, and fresh parsley.
3. **Make the Dressing:**
   - In a small bowl, whisk together the extra-virgin olive oil, red wine vinegar, dried oregano, salt, and pepper.

4. **Dress the Salad:**
   - Pour the dressing over the chickpea and vegetable mixture. Toss gently to coat all ingredients evenly.
5. **Add Feta (Optional):**
   - If using feta cheese, crumble it over the salad and toss gently.
6. **Chill (Optional):**
   - Refrigerate the salad for at least 30 minutes to allow the flavors to meld. This step is optional but enhances the taste.
7. **Garnish and Serve:**
   - Before serving, garnish with Kalamata olives if desired. Serve chilled or at room temperature.

Benefits:
1. **Protein-Rich:**
   - Chickpeas are an excellent source of plant-based protein, making this salad a satisfying and nutritious option.
2. **Rich in Vitamins and Antioxidants:**
   - Tomatoes and cucumbers contribute vitamins, minerals, and antioxidants to support overall health.
3. **Heart-Healthy Fats:**
   - Olive oil provides monounsaturated fats, which are beneficial for heart health.

4. **Digestive Health:**
   - The fiber in chickpeas and vegetables promotes healthy digestion.

Application:

1. **Quick and Healthy Lunch:**
   - Chickpea and Tomato Salad is perfect for a quick and healthy lunch, offering a good balance of protein, fiber, and vitamins.
2. **Side Dish:**
   - Serve it as a refreshing side dish alongside grilled chicken, fish, or your favorite protein.
3. **Potluck or Picnic Contribution:**
   - Bring this salad to potlucks, picnics, or barbecues as a flavorful and nutritious contribution.
4. **Mediterranean Meal:**
   - Include this salad in a Mediterranean-inspired meal with other dishes like hummus, tzatziki, and grilled vegetables.
5. **Meal Prep:**
   - Prepare a batch for meal prep and enjoy it throughout the week as a convenient and satisfying option.

Baked Cod with Lemon and Herbs

Ingredients:
- 4 cod fillets (6 oz each)
- 2 tablespoons olive oil
- 2 tablespoons fresh lemon juice
- 2 cloves garlic, minced
- 1 teaspoon dried oregano
- 1 teaspoon dried thyme
- Salt and pepper to taste
- Lemon slices for garnish
- Fresh parsley, chopped, for garnish

Instructions:
1. **Preheat the Oven:**
   - Preheat your oven to 400°F (200°C).
2. **Prepare the Cod Fillets:**
   - Pat the cod fillets dry with paper towels. Place them in a baking dish lined with parchment paper or lightly greased.
3. **Make the Marinade:**
   - In a small bowl, whisk together the olive oil, fresh lemon juice, minced garlic, dried oregano, dried thyme, salt, and pepper.
4. **Marinate the Cod:**
   - Pour the marinade over the cod fillets, ensuring they are well-

coated on all sides. Let them marinate for 15-30 minutes.

5. **Bake the Cod:**
   - Bake the cod in the preheated oven for 15-20 minutes or until the fish flakes easily with a fork. The cooking time may vary depending on the thickness of the fillets.
6. **Broil for Crispy Top (Optional):**
   - If you desire a crispy top, broil the cod for an additional 2-3 minutes until the top is golden brown.
7. **Garnish and Serve:**
   - Remove the cod from the oven. Garnish with lemon slices and chopped fresh parsley. Serve immediately.

Benefits:
1. **High-Quality Protein:**
   - Cod is a lean source of high-quality protein, essential for muscle health and overall well-being.
2. **Heart-Healthy Fats:**
   - Olive oil provides monounsaturated fats, which are beneficial for heart health.
3. **Rich in Omega-3 Fatty Acids:**
   - Cod is a good source of omega-3 fatty acids, promoting cardiovascular health.

4. **Low in Calories:**
   - Baked cod is a low-calorie option, making it suitable for those watching their calorie intake.

Application:
1. **Healthy Dinner Option:**
   - Baked Cod with Lemon and Herbs is a quick and healthy option for a satisfying dinner.
2. **Date Night Meal:**
   - Impress your guests with this flavorful and elegant dish, perfect for a date night or special occasion.
3. **Meal Prep:**
   - Prepare multiple fillets and store them in individual portions for convenient meal prep throughout the week.
4. **Pair with Sides:**
   - Serve the cod with your favorite sides such as roasted vegetables, quinoa, or a fresh salad for a well-balanced meal.
5. **Lemon-Herb Variation:**
   - Customize the recipe by experimenting with different herbs or adding lemon zest for extra citrus flavor.

Quinoa-Stuffed Bell Peppers

Ingredients:

- 4 large bell peppers, halved and seeds removed
- 1 cup quinoa, rinsed
- 2 cups vegetable broth or water
- 1 can (15 oz) black beans, drained and rinsed
- 1 cup corn kernels (fresh, frozen, or canned)
- 1 cup cherry tomatoes, diced
- 1/2 red onion, finely chopped
- 2 cloves garlic, minced
- 1 teaspoon ground cumin
- 1 teaspoon chili powder
- 1/2 teaspoon smoked paprika
- 1 cup shredded cheese (cheddar, Monterey Jack, or your choice)
- 2 tablespoons olive oil
- Salt and pepper to taste
- Fresh cilantro or parsley for garnish (optional)

Instructions:

1. **Preheat the Oven:**
   - Preheat your oven to 375°F (190°C).
2. **Cook Quinoa:**
   - In a saucepan, combine quinoa and vegetable broth or water. Bring to a boil, then reduce heat to low, cover,

and simmer for 15-20 minutes or until quinoa is cooked and liquid is absorbed.

3. **Prepare Bell Peppers:**
   - Cut the bell peppers in half lengthwise and remove seeds and membranes. Place them in a baking dish.

4. **Sauté Aromatics:**
   - In a large skillet, heat olive oil over medium heat. Add minced garlic and chopped red onion. Sauté until the onion is translucent and fragrant.

5. **Add Vegetables:**
   - Add black beans, corn, cherry tomatoes, ground cumin, chili powder, smoked paprika, salt, and pepper to the skillet. Cook for 5-7 minutes, stirring occasionally.

6. **Combine Quinoa and Vegetables:**
   - In a large bowl, combine the cooked quinoa with the sautéed vegetable mixture. Mix well.

7. **Stuff Bell Peppers:**
   - Stuff each bell pepper half with the quinoa and vegetable mixture, pressing it down gently.

8. **Bake:**
   - Sprinkle shredded cheese over the stuffed bell peppers. Cover the

baking dish with aluminum foil and bake in the preheated oven for 25-30 minutes or until the peppers are tender.

9. **Broil (Optional):**
   - If you desire a golden brown top, uncover the baking dish and broil for an additional 2-3 minutes until the cheese is bubbly and slightly crispy.
10. **Garnish and Serve:**
    - Garnish with fresh cilantro or parsley if desired. Serve the quinoa-stuffed bell peppers hot.

Benefits:
1. **Plant-Based Protein:**
   - Quinoa and black beans provide a combination of plant-based proteins, making this dish suitable for vegetarians and vegans.
2. **Fiber-Rich:**
   - Quinoa, black beans, and vegetables contribute dietary fiber, promoting digestive health.
3. **Nutrient-Dense:**
   - Bell peppers are rich in vitamins A and C, while quinoa provides essential amino acids.
4. **Versatile:**
   - This dish is versatile and can be customized with various vegetables

and spices according to taste preferences.

Application:

1. **Vegetarian Main Course:**
   - Quinoa-Stuffed Bell Peppers make for a hearty and satisfying vegetarian main course.

2. **Meal Prep:**
   - Prepare a batch for meal prep and enjoy them throughout the week for quick and convenient meals.

3. **Side Dish:**
   - Serve as a flavorful and nutritious side dish alongside grilled chicken, fish, or your favorite protein.

4. **Make-Ahead Dinner:**
   - Prepare the stuffed peppers in advance and bake them just before serving for a quick and easy dinner option.

5. **Party or Potluck Dish:**
   - Bring this dish to parties or potlucks as a crowd-pleasing and visually appealing option.

Spinach and Berry Smoothie

Ingredients:
- 1 cup fresh spinach leaves
- 1/2 cup frozen mixed berries (strawberries, blueberries, raspberries)
- 1 banana, peeled
- 1/2 cup Greek yogurt (plain or flavored)
- 1/2 cup almond milk (or your preferred milk)
- 1 tablespoon chia seeds
- 1 tablespoon honey or maple syrup (optional for sweetness)
- Ice cubes (optional)

Instructions:
1. **Prepare Ingredients:**
   - Wash the fresh spinach leaves and peel the banana.
2. **Blend Spinach and Liquid:**
   - In a blender, combine the fresh spinach and almond milk. Blend until the spinach is well incorporated and the mixture is smooth.
3. **Add Berries and Banana:**
   - Add the frozen mixed berries and peeled banana to the blender.
4. **Include Greek Yogurt and Chia Seeds:**
   - Spoon in the Greek yogurt and add chia seeds to the blender.

5. **Sweeten (Optional):**
   - If you desire additional sweetness, add honey or maple syrup to taste.
6. **Blend until Smooth:**
   - Blend all the ingredients until smooth and creamy. If the consistency is too thick, you can add more almond milk.
7. **Adjust Texture:**
   - If desired, add ice cubes and blend again until the smoothie reaches your preferred consistency.
8. **Serve:**
   - Pour the Spinach and Berry Smoothie into a glass and serve immediately.

Benefits:
1. **Nutrient-Rich:**
   - Spinach is a powerhouse of nutrients, including vitamins A, C, and K, iron, and fiber.
2. **Antioxidants:**
   - Berries are rich in antioxidants, which help combat oxidative stress in the body.
3. **Protein and Probiotics:**
   - Greek yogurt provides a good source of protein and probiotics, supporting gut health.

4. **Omega-3 Fatty Acids:**
   - Chia seeds contribute omega-3 fatty acids, promoting heart and brain health.

Application:

1. **Breakfast Option:**
   - Enjoy the Spinach and Berry Smoothie as a nutritious and energizing breakfast option.
2. **Post-Workout Refuel:**
   - The combination of protein, carbohydrates, and nutrients makes this smoothie an excellent choice for post-workout recovery.
3. **Snack Time:**
   - Have this smoothie as a healthy and satisfying snack between meals.
4. **Kids' Friendly:**
   - It's a great way to sneak in greens for kids while offering a naturally sweet and flavorful drink.
5. **Meal Replacement:**
   - Use this smoothie as a meal replacement for a quick and nourishing option on busy days.

Sweet Potato and Lentil Soup

Ingredients:

- 1 cup dry green or brown lentils, rinsed and drained
- 2 large sweet potatoes, peeled and diced
- 1 onion, diced
- 2 carrots, peeled and chopped
- 2 celery stalks, chopped
- 3 cloves garlic, minced
- 1 teaspoon ground cumin
- 1 teaspoon ground coriander
- 1/2 teaspoon smoked paprika
- 1/4 teaspoon cayenne pepper (optional, for added heat)
- 6 cups vegetable broth
- 1 can (14 oz) diced tomatoes, undrained
- 2 tablespoons olive oil
- Salt and pepper to taste
- Fresh cilantro or parsley for garnish (optional)
- Greek yogurt or coconut milk for serving (optional)

Instructions:

1. **Prepare Lentils:**
   - Rinse the lentils under cold water and drain.
2. **Sauté Vegetables:**
   - In a large pot, heat olive oil over medium heat. Add diced onion, carrots, celery, and minced garlic.

Sauté until the vegetables are softened.

3. **Add Spices:**
   - Stir in ground cumin, ground coriander, smoked paprika, and cayenne pepper (if using). Cook for an additional 1-2 minutes to toast the spices.

4. **Combine Lentils and Sweet Potatoes:**
   - Add the rinsed lentils, diced sweet potatoes, vegetable broth, and diced tomatoes (with their juice) to the pot. Season with salt and pepper.

5. **Simmer:**
   - Bring the soup to a boil, then reduce the heat to low, cover, and simmer for about 25-30 minutes or until the lentils and sweet potatoes are tender.

6. **Blend (Optional):**
   - For a creamier consistency, use an immersion blender to partially blend the soup. Alternatively, transfer a portion of the soup to a blender and blend until smooth, then return it to the pot.

7. **Adjust Seasoning:**
   - Taste the soup and adjust the seasoning with salt and pepper as needed.

8. **Serve:**
   - Ladle the Sweet Potato and Lentil Soup into bowls. Garnish with fresh cilantro or parsley if desired. Serve with a dollop of Greek yogurt or a drizzle of coconut milk if desired.

Benefits:
1. **Rich in Fiber:**
   - Lentils and sweet potatoes are high in fiber, promoting digestive health and providing a feeling of fullness.
2. **Vitamins and Minerals:**
   - Sweet potatoes are rich in vitamins A and C, while lentils provide essential nutrients like iron and folate.
3. **Protein Source:**
   - Lentils contribute plant-based protein, making this soup a nutritious option for vegetarians and vegans.
4. **Anti-Inflammatory:**
   - Spices like cumin, coriander, and turmeric have anti-inflammatory properties.

Application:
1. **Hearty Winter Meal:**
   - Sweet Potato and Lentil Soup is a comforting and hearty option, especially during colder months.

2. **Meal Prep:**
   - Prepare a batch and store it in individual portions for convenient meal prep throughout the week.
3. **Lunch or Dinner Option:**
   - Enjoy the soup as a satisfying lunch or dinner option, paired with crusty bread or a side salad.
4. **Freeze for Later:**
   - Freeze portions of the soup for future quick and easy meals.
5. **Vegan-Friendly:**
   - Serve the soup as a vegan-friendly option by omitting any dairy-based toppings.

Salmon and Avocado Wrap

Ingredients:

- 2 salmon fillets (about 6 oz each), grilled or baked
- 2 large whole-grain or spinach tortillas
- 1 ripe avocado, sliced
- 1 cup mixed greens (arugula, spinach, or your choice)
- 1/4 cup red onion, thinly sliced
- 1/4 cup cucumber, julienned
- 2 tablespoons Greek yogurt or sour cream
- 1 tablespoon fresh dill, chopped
- 1 tablespoon capers (optional)
- 1 tablespoon olive oil
- Salt and pepper to taste
- Lemon wedges for serving

Instructions:

1. **Prepare Salmon:**
   - Grill or bake the salmon fillets until fully cooked. Season with salt and pepper to taste.
2. **Assemble Wrap:**
   - Lay out the tortillas on a flat surface. Place a portion of mixed greens in the center of each tortilla.
3. **Add Salmon and Avocado:**
   - Flake the grilled or baked salmon and distribute it evenly over the mixed greens. Top with sliced avocado.

4. **Include Vegetables:**
   - Sprinkle thinly sliced red onion and julienned cucumber over the salmon and avocado.
5. **Prepare Yogurt Sauce:**
   - In a small bowl, mix Greek yogurt or sour cream with chopped fresh dill. This will be the sauce for the wrap.
6. **Drizzle with Sauce:**
   - Drizzle the yogurt sauce over the ingredients in each wrap.
7. **Add Optional Ingredients:**
   - If using capers, sprinkle them over the wraps. Capers add a briny and flavorful touch.
8. **Drizzle with Olive Oil:**
   - Drizzle a bit of olive oil over the wraps for added richness and flavor.
9. **Fold and Serve:**
   - Fold the sides of the tortillas over the filling to create a wrap. Secure with toothpicks if needed. Cut in half if desired and serve with lemon wedges on the side.

Benefits:

1. **Omega-3 Fatty Acids:**
   - Salmon is rich in omega-3 fatty acids, which are beneficial for heart and brain health.

2. **Healthy Fats:**
   - Avocado provides monounsaturated fats, contributing to heart health.
3. **Protein-Rich:**
   - Salmon is a excellent source of high-quality protein, supporting muscle health.
4. **Nutrient-Dense Vegetables:**
   - The wrap includes nutrient-dense vegetables like mixed greens, red onion, and cucumber.

Application:
1. **Quick and Healthy Lunch:**
   - The Salmon and Avocado Wrap is a quick and healthy option for a satisfying lunch.
2. **Post-Workout Meal:**
   - Enjoy this wrap as a nutritious post-workout meal to replenish protein and healthy fats.
3. **Outdoor Picnic or BBQ:**
   - Pack these wraps for an outdoor picnic or barbecue, as they are easy to transport and assemble on-site.
4. **Light Dinner Option:**
   - Serve the wraps as a light and flavorful dinner option, accompanied by a side salad.
5. **Customizable:**
   - Customize the wraps by adding your favorite herbs, spices, or

additional vegetables for extra flavor and nutrition.

Quinoa Salad with Roasted Vegetables

Ingredients:

- 1 cup quinoa, rinsed
- 2 cups water or vegetable broth
- 1 red bell pepper, diced
- 1 yellow bell pepper, diced
- 1 zucchini, diced
- 1 cup cherry tomatoes, halved
- 1 red onion, thinly sliced
- 3 tablespoons olive oil
- 2 cloves garlic, minced
- 1 teaspoon dried oregano
- 1 teaspoon dried thyme
- Salt and pepper to taste
- 1/4 cup feta cheese, crumbled (optional)
- 2 tablespoons balsamic vinegar
- Fresh basil or parsley for garnish

Instructions:

1. **Cook Quinoa:**
   - In a medium saucepan, combine quinoa and water or vegetable broth. Bring to a boil, then reduce heat to low, cover, and simmer for 15-20 minutes or until quinoa is cooked and liquid is absorbed. Fluff with a fork.
2. **Preheat Oven:**
   - Preheat the oven to 400°F (200°C).

3. **Prepare Vegetables:**
   - In a large mixing bowl, combine diced red and yellow bell peppers, zucchini, cherry tomatoes, and sliced red onion.
4. **Make Roasting Marinade:**
   - In a small bowl, whisk together olive oil, minced garlic, dried oregano, dried thyme, salt, and pepper. Pour the marinade over the vegetables and toss to coat evenly.
5. **Roast Vegetables:**
   - Spread the vegetables in a single layer on a baking sheet. Roast in the preheated oven for 20-25 minutes or until the vegetables are tender and slightly caramelized. Stir halfway through for even roasting.
6. **Combine Quinoa and Vegetables:**
   - In a large serving bowl, combine the cooked quinoa and roasted vegetables. Toss gently to mix.
7. **Add Feta (Optional):**
   - If using, sprinkle crumbled feta cheese over the quinoa and vegetables.
8. **Drizzle with Balsamic Vinegar:**
   - Drizzle balsamic vinegar over the salad and toss once more to combine.

9. **Garnish and Serve:**
   - Garnish with fresh basil or parsley. Serve the Quinoa Salad with Roasted Vegetables warm or at room temperature.

Benefits:
1. **Protein and Fiber:**
   - Quinoa is a complete protein source, and both quinoa and vegetables contribute dietary fiber, promoting satiety and digestive health.
2. **Rich in Antioxidants:**
   - Bell peppers, tomatoes, and zucchini are rich in antioxidants, which help protect cells from damage.
3. **Heart-Healthy Fats:**
   - Olive oil provides monounsaturated fats, contributing to heart health.
4. **Vitamins and Minerals:**
   - Vegetables offer a variety of essential vitamins and minerals for overall well-being.

Application:
1. **Main Course or Side Dish:**
   - Serve the Quinoa Salad with Roasted Vegetables as a satisfying main course or as a flavorful side dish.

2. **Meal Prep:**
   - Prepare a batch and store it in individual portions for convenient meal prep throughout the week.
3. **Potluck or BBQ Contribution:**
   - Bring this salad to potlucks, barbecues, or gatherings as a visually appealing and nutritious contribution.
4. **Vegan Option:**
   - Omit the feta cheese for a vegan-friendly version of this salad.
5. **Customizable:**
   - Customize the recipe by adding your favorite herbs, nuts, or additional vegetables to suit your taste preferences.

CONCLUSION

Upon the completion of this emotional trip through "Fix It and Forget It Breast Cancer Recipes," we would like to send our best wishes for well-being, resilience, and sustenance. This book is a celebration of resiliency, community, and the restorative power of food—it is much more than just a list of recipes.

The journey through breast cancer may be difficult, but taking care of oneself may be a simple yet powerful act. These recipes are thoughtfully and carefully prepared, taking into account the special requirements that develop during treatment and recuperation.

The "Fix It and Forget It" method welcomes the notion that healthy eating doesn't have to be difficult, freeing you to concentrate on what really counts: your wellbeing.

I hope these recipes turn into a dependable partner that brings happiness, warmth, and nourishment. Remind yourself that you have company on this road.

Let these dishes serve as a reminder that every meal made with love aids in the healing process, whether you are the one dealing with breast cancer or you are supporting a loved one.

I'm wishing you peaceful moments, delectable food, and the fortitude to confront every day head-on. May your table serve as a gathering spot and a place for healing, and may your kitchen be a haven of comfort.

Accept the coziness and ease of "Fix It and Forget It Breast Cancer Recipes," from our hearts to yours. You are surrounded by people who genuinely care about your well-being, yet you underestimate your strength.